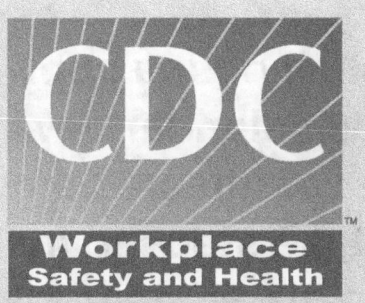

Evaluation of Prostate Cancer, Diesel Exhaust Exposures, and Radio Frequency Exposures Among Employees at a Rail Yard – Alabama

Marie A. de Perio, MD
Kenneth W. Fent, PhD

Health Hazard Evaluation Report
HETA 2011-0045-3149
December 2011

DEPARTMENT OF HEALTH AND HUMAN SERVICES
Centers for Disease Control and Prevention

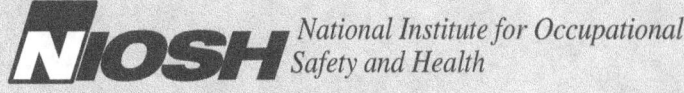 National Institute for Occupational Safety and Health

CONTENTS

REPORT

APPENDIX

ACKNOWLEDGMENTS

ABBREVIATIONS

$\mu g/m^3$	Micrograms per cubic meter
μm	Micrometer
ACGIH®	American Conference of Governmental Industrial Hygienists
ANSI	American National Standards Institute
CFR	Code of Federal Regulations
CO	Carbon monoxide
FCC	Federal Communications Commission
GHz	Gigahertz
HHE	Health hazard evaluation
IARC	International Agency for Research on Cancer
ICNIRP	International Commission on Non-Ionizing Radiation Protection
IEEE	Institute for Electrical and Electronics Engineers
kHz	Kilohertz
Lpm	Liters per minute
MDC	Minimum detectable concentration
MHz	Megahertz
m^3	Cubic meter
mm	Millimeter
MQC	Minimum quantifiable concentration
mW/cm^2	Milliwatts per square centimeter
NA	Not applicable
ND	None detected
NAICS	North American Industry Classification System
NIOSH	National Institute for Occupational Safety and Health
NO	Nitric oxide
NO_2	Nitrogen dioxide
OEL	Occupational exposure limit
OSHA	Occupational Safety and Health Administration
Particles/cm^3	Particles per cubic centimeter
PEL	Permissible exposure limit
ppm	Parts per million
RCL	Remote control locomotive
REL	Recommended exposure limit
SO_2	Sulfur dioxide
STEL	Short-term exposure limit
TLV®	Threshold limit value
TWA	Time-weighted average
WEEL™	Workplace environmental exposure level

The National Institute for Occupational Safety and Health received a confidential employee request for a health hazard evaluation at a rail yard in Alabama. The employees submitted the request because of concerns about prostate cancer and exposures to diesel exhaust, radio frequencies, and vibration.

What NIOSH Did

- We interviewed employees reported to have been diagnosed with prostate cancer.

- We visited the rail yard in June 2011.

- We observed work practices and interviewed 33 transportation department employees.

- We sampled the air for components of diesel exhaust.

- We measured radio frequency power density levels from the remote control locomotive (RCL) devices and two-way radios.

What NIOSH Found

- The number of prostate cancer cases among employees at the rail yard was not unusual.

- Prostate cancer among employees was likely not the result of working at the rail yard.

- The components of diesel exhaust that we measured in air were generally low.

- It is unlikely that transportation department employees were overexposed to radio frequencies.

- Inconsistent use of hearing protection by employees was observed and reported.

What Managers Can Do

- Take additional air samples for elemental carbon to assess exposure to diesel exhaust. Sample the positions with the highest exposure levels noted in this report.

- Include more detailed education on radio frequencies during the RCL device training for operators.

- Make sure that employees know to whom they should report work-related health problems.

- Post signs in the hump yard that state hearing protection is required in that area.

- Make push-in earplugs more accessible to all employees or provide communication earmuffs that can be worn throughout the work shift.

- Have rail yard employees' hearing tested annually.

What Employees Can Do

- Learn more about the risk factors of cancer and what you can do to lower your risk.

- Make sure that the health information you find is reliable, unbiased, and up-to-date.

Summary

NIOSH investigators examined the occurrence of prostate cancer among transportation department employees at a rail yard and their exposures to diesel exhaust, radio frequencies, and vibration. The number of prostate cancer cases reported among employees was not unusual. The cancers were not likely to have an occupational cause. Exposures to diesel exhaust were below the applicable OEL for all but one employee. According to our measurements, employees were unlikely to be overexposed to radio frequencies.

In January 2011, we received a confidential HHE request from employees of a rail yard in Alabama. The request concerned the occurrence of prostate cancer among transportation department employees and their exposures to diesel exhaust, radio frequencies, and vibration.

Prior to our visit, we interviewed by phone 8 of 12 current or former surviving employees reported to have been diagnosed with prostate cancer. We also reviewed the railroad company's records and other information related to employees' exposures to diesel exhaust, radio frequencies, and vibration. During our on-site evaluation in June 2011, we interviewed 33 transportation department employees and observed work processes, practices, and workplace conditions. We also sampled the air for components of diesel exhaust and measured radio frequency power density levels from the RCL devices and two-way radios. We did not evaluate vibration because previous studies by the railroad company indicated low vibration magnitudes for employees riding locomotives.

The number of prostate cancer cases identified among current and former employees at the rail yard did not appear to be unusual. The prostate cancer reported among workers was likely not the result of working at the rail yard. While most of the 33 interviewed employees reported experiencing at least one health symptom (such as fatigue, headache, runny nose, or congestion) while working, the symptoms can be attributed to various etiologies including heat and underlying seasonal allergies and asthma. Personal exposures to elemental carbon from diesel exhaust were below the applicable OEL for all but one employee. Other sources of elemental carbon may have contributed to the one overexposure, but this requires further evaluation. Our measurements of power density levels suggest that the transportation department employees were unlikely to be overexposed to radio frequencies.

We recommend that the railroad company conduct additional air sampling for elemental carbon, focusing on the positions for which we measured the highest personal air concentrations identified in this report. The company should also provide more detailed education on radio frequencies during the initial and refresher RCL device training for operators. In addition, employees should learn more about known cancer risk factors and what they can do to minimize those risk factors.

Keywords: NAICS 482111 (Line-Haul Railroads), prostate cancer, cancer cluster, railroad, diesel exhaust, vibration, radiofrequency, elemental carbon, nitric oxide, nitrogen dioxide

This page left intentionally blank

INTRODUCTION

In January 2011, NIOSH received an HHE request from employees of a rail yard in Alabama. The request concerned prostate cancer among the transportation department employees at the rail yard and their exposures to diesel exhaust, radio frequencies, and vibration.

Prior to our visit, we interviewed by phone current and former employees reported to have been diagnosed with prostate cancer and reviewed the railroad company's records and other information related to employees' exposures to diesel exhaust, radio frequencies, and vibration. We conducted an on-site evaluation in June 2011 where we observed work processes, practices, and workplace conditions and interviewed transportation department employees. We also sampled the air for components of diesel exhaust and measured radio frequency power density levels from the RCL devices and two-way radios.

Rail Yard Operations

At the time of our HHE, the railroad company provided rail-based transportation services throughout the United States and Canada. The company operated track structures as well as rail yards and terminals. These rail yards and terminals served as classification facilities where railcars were received, sorted, and placed onto new outbound trains. The company operated 36 rail yards within its system.

The rail yard in Alabama employed more than 500 people in its engineering, mechanical, and transportation departments. The approximately 400 transportation department employees were responsible for the safe and efficient operation of trains and the movement of customer freight from one destination to another. Within the transportation department, freight conductors (also called yard foremen) supervised train crews, coordinated switch engine crews, and placed cars to facilitate the loading and unloading and the makeup and breakdown of trains in the yard. Trainmen (also called switchmen or brakemen) switched the railcars and assisted with train operations; engineers operated the locomotives.

RCL devices, worn around the waist by transportation department employees, were used to remotely control locomotives to assist in the classification of railcars (Figure 1). Classification was performed at the south, bowl, and hump yards. In the hump yard, cars were pushed up the hump and then released to be sorted by the force of gravity. Classification in the other areas of the rail yard was accomplished on level ground using locomotives to move cars onto different tracks.

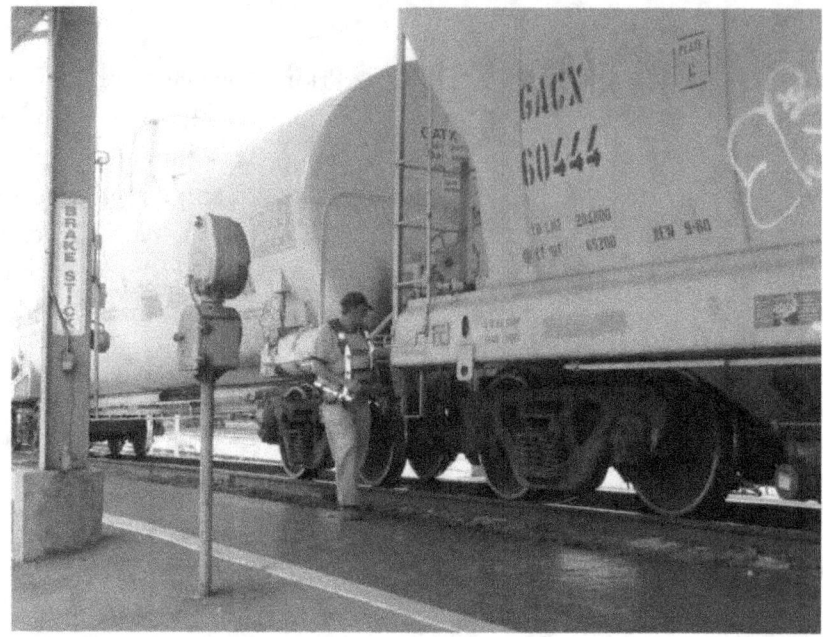

Figure 1. Freight conductor using the RCL device to direct rail cars up the hump to be released and sorted by gravity.

Cancer and Prostate Cancer

Cancer is a group of diseases characterized by the uncontrolled growth and spread of abnormal cells. There are many different types of cancer, and each cancer has its own set of causes, some known and some not yet discovered. Approximately one third of cancer deaths are caused by tobacco use and another third are related to obesity, physical inactivity, and poor nutrition [American Cancer Society 2011].

About 1,596,670 new cancer cases are expected to be diagnosed in the United States in 2011, while about 571,950 people were expected to die of cancer in 2010 [American Cancer Society 2011]. In the United States, the lifetime risk of developing cancer is 1 in 2 in men and 1 in 3 in women [American Cancer Society 2011].

Prostate cancer is a type of cancer that starts in the prostate, a walnut-sized organ located just below the bladder and in front of the rectum in men. It produces fluid that makes up a part of semen. Prostate cancer is the most frequently diagnosed cancer in men, and an estimated 240,890 new cases of prostate cancer will occur in the United States in 2011 [American Cancer Society

2011]. One in six men will be diagnosed with prostate cancer during his lifetime. Prostate cancer is the second-leading cause of cancer death in men, with an estimated 33,720 deaths in 2011 [American Cancer Society 2011]. One in 36 men will die of prostate cancer.

Early prostate cancer usually has no symptoms. When they occur, symptoms include difficulty in starting urination, weak or interrupted flow of urine, difficulty in emptying the bladder completely, pain or burning during urination, blood in the urine or semen, frequent urination especially at night, painful ejaculation, and pain in the back, hips, or pelvis that doesn't go away.

The only well-established risk factors for prostate cancer are age ≥ 50 years, African-American race, and having a family history of the disease [American Cancer Society 2011]. No occupational or environmental risk factors for prostate cancer are known. Rail transport workers have not consistently been shown to have a statistically significant excess of diagnosed prostate cancer [Aronson et al. 1996; Krstev et al. 1998a; Krstev et al. 1998b].

Diesel Exhaust

Diesel exhaust is a mixture of gases and particles. The particulate fraction of diesel exhaust is composed of microscopic cores of elemental carbon, onto which are adsorbed organic carbon compounds [NIOSH 1988; OSHA 1988]. Diesel particulate matter consists of fine particles (0–2.5 μm in aerodynamic diameter), including a high number of ultrafine particles (< 0.1 μm in aerodynamic diameter) [Wichmann 2007]. Some of the main gases in diesel exhaust are oxides of nitrogen, sulfur, and carbon [NIOSH 1988; OSHA 1988]. Exposure to diesel exhaust has been associated with acute and chronic respiratory effects and lung cancer [EPA 2002]. The Appendix provides more information about diesel exhaust exposures and health effects.

Air sampling for diesel exhaust constituents had not been conducted at this rail yard, but management representatives from the railroad company did provide us with elemental carbon measurements collected at their other rail yards. A total of 188 personal air samples had been collected from transportation department employees for the analysis of elemental carbon. All were below the California Department of Health Services OEL of 20 µg/m³ [CDHS 2002]. However, because other rail yards may have different workplace and environmental conditions, we determined that conducting air sampling for diesel exhaust constituents at this rail yard was necessary.

Radio Frequency

Electromagnetic waves that have frequencies ranging from 3 kHz to 300 GHz are considered radio frequencies [FCC 1999]. According to information provided to us by the manufacturer, Cattron Group International (Sparpsville, Pennsylvania), the Accuspeed™ RCL devices operate at 450–470 MHz. The two-way radios (Nexedge NX-200/300, Kenwood USA, Long Beach, California) operate at 136–174 MHz. The RCL devices (2 watts or less) and two-way radios (5 watts) have relatively low power. The RCL device transmits on a shared time slot and has stationary repeaters that allow it to transmit over longer distances.

Cattron Group International also gave us the specification sheet they used to calculate the power density emanating from the RCL device. The variables and formula they used to calculate the power density were appropriate. Their calculated power density (0.11 mW/cm²) was 10% of the applicable ICNIRP OEL [ICNIRP 1998], which is the most conservative OEL. However, because actual measurements can vary from calculations, and other radio frequency sources (two-way radios) existed at the rail yard, we determined that it was necessary to collect radio frequency measurements when employees were operating RCL devices and two-way radios.

Radio frequencies do not have enough energy to displace electrons from atoms or molecules (or cause genetic mutations) and, therefore, are considered non-ionizing radiation [FCC 1999]. The primary effect of concern from radio frequencies is the heating of biological tissue [FCC 1999]. The Appendix provides more information about radio frequency exposures and health effects.

Vibration

Vibration above recommended exposure limits has been associated with changes in the tendons, muscles, bones, joints, and nervous system. Whole-body vibration can cause fatigue, insomnia, stomach problems, headache, and shakiness shortly after or during exposure [Canada Center for Occupational Health and Safety 2011].

INTRODUCTION (CONTINUED)

Management representatives from the railroad company gave us reports from two locomotive vibration studies that were conducted by Applied Safety and Ergonomics, Inc. (Ann Arbor, Michigan). Both studies were comprehensive and found whole-body vibration magnitudes below the "Health Guidance Caution Zone" from ANSI S3.18-2002 [ANSI 2002]. On the basis of these findings, we decided not to further evaluate vibration from riding locomotives at the rail yard.

ASSESSMENT

The purpose of our HHE was to (1) investigate prostate cancer and assess health symptoms among transportation department employees through confidential medical interviews, (2) characterize diesel exhaust exposures to transportation department employees, (3) measure power density levels from radio frequency emitting devices used by transportation department employees, and (4) evaluate other potential hazards and health and safety policies at the rail yard.

Confidential Medical Interviews

Prior to our visit, we were given a list of 13 current and former employees reportedly diagnosed with prostate cancer since 1999. One employee had died. We contacted the 10 employees for whom we were provided contact information and interviewed them by phone. During these interviews, we asked them about their age at diagnosis, their personal risk factors for prostate cancer, and their work history.

During our visit to the rail yard on June 13–15, 2011, we held confidential medical interviews with first, second, and third shift transportation department employees to discuss their work history, pertinent medical history including diagnoses of cancer, symptoms experienced during work, and other health and workplace concerns. All transportation department employees working in the hump, bowl, and south yards at the time of the interviews were invited to participate. An additional three transportation department employees working in other locations within the rail yard asked to participate. During these interviews, we also discussed the differences between ionizing and non-ionizing radiation and their potential to cause cancer. We explained that the radio frequencies emitted from the RCL devices were of low frequency, considered non-ionizing radiation, and had not been established as a cause of cancer in adults. We also discussed known risk factors for prostate cancer and informed employees what they could do to prevent cancer.

Assessment of Diesel Exhaust and Radio Frequency Exposures

We collected work-shift personal breathing zone and area air samples for the following constituents of diesel exhaust: elemental carbon particles; "fine" particles (0.01 μm to >1 μm); and NO, NO_2, SO_2, and CO gases. Table 1 provides a summary of the elemental carbon sampling methods, and Table 2 provides a summary of the other direct-reading sampling methods we used.

Table 1. Summary of the elemental carbon air sampling methods

Analyte	Sampling Media/Equipment	Flow Rate (Lpm)	Analytical Method†	Number of Samples	
				Personal	Area
Total elemental carbon	25-mm quartz fiber filter, open face	4	NIOSH 5040	11	3
Respirable elemental carbon	25-mm quartz fiber filter with GK 2.69 cyclone (BGI Incorporated, Waltham, Massachusetts)*	4	NIOSH 5040	5	3

*Includes specially designed screw-in adapter for 25-mm cassettes developed by Dr. Eileen Birch at NIOSH.
†NIOSH Manual of Analytical Methods [NIOSH 2011].

Table 2. Summary of the direct-reading air sampling methods

Analyte	Sampling Media/Equipment	Number of Samples	
		Personal	Area
NO	GasAlert single gas meters (BW	6	NA
NO_2	Technologies, Arlington, Texas) set to record	6	NA
SO_2	every 5 seconds	6	NA
CO		6	NA
Fine particles (0.01 μm to > 1 μm)	Condensation particle counter (TSI Incorporated, Shoreview, Minnesota) set to record every second	NA	7
Radio frequency power density	HI-4460 broadband isotropic field meter (ETS-Lindgren, Cedar Park, Texas) set to record every half second	NA	5

Personal sampling was performed on 11 employees over a 2-day period. All 11 employees wore total elemental carbon samplers. Of these employees, five also wore respirable elemental carbon samplers on the opposite sides of their bodies relative to the total elemental carbon samplers, and the other six employees wore NO, NO_2, SO_2, and CO meters on various body locations. Paired total and respirable elemental carbon area air samples were collected in three different locations of the rail yard. Most of the personal and area air samples were collected over the entire work shift (approximately 8 hours). The cyclone in the respirable dust sampler had a cut point of 4.2 μm and was used to exclude any potential contribution of elemental carbon from non-combustion sources, such as coal dust in the rail cars. The direct-reading fine particle measurements were made to determine if sources of fine particles other than diesel exhaust from the locomotive engines existed at or near the rail yard.

We collected only a few radio frequency power density measurements near employees while they operated the RCL devices or two-way radios. Our goal was to determine whether a more comprehensive evaluation of radio frequency exposure was needed at the rail yard.

All measurements we collected were compared to applicable OELs. These OELs are listed in the Results section. The Appendix provides more information about these OELs.

Observation of Work Practices

During our visit to the rail yard, we observed work practices among transportation department employees in the south, hump, and bowl yards. We specifically observed employees' adherence to measures that reduced the potential for heat stress and adherence to the use of hearing protection.

Interviews with Employees Diagnosed with Prostate Cancer

We interviewed by phone 10 of the 12 living current or former employees reportedly diagnosed with prostate cancer since 1999. One employee did not have a diagnosis of prostate cancer and another employee, who confirmed a diagnosis of prostate cancer, worked at a different rail yard.

The remaining eight employees all confirmed diagnoses of prostate cancer. Five were Caucasian, and three were African American. The median age at diagnosis was 54 years (range: 50–60 years). Years of diagnosis ranged from 1999–2009. Three employees reported a family history of prostate cancer, and four reported they were a former or current smoker.

Of the eight employees, five were retired, and three were currently working at the rail yard. Two were diagnosed with prostate cancer after retirement from the railroad company. Three worked as engineers, and five worked as conductors/trainmen. The median number of years between the start of their employment at the railroad company and diagnosis was 31 years, with a range of 28–41 years.

Onsite Interviews with Employees

All 33 invited employees participated in the interviews. All were male. One employee was African American and the other 32 were Caucasian. The median age of the 33 employees was 39 years (range: 25–59 years). Work characteristics of the 33 interviewed employees are shown in Table 3.

The median years worked at the railroad company was 9 (range: 1–38 years). The median number of years worked at the rail yard was 8 (range: 1–35 years). Thirty (91%) employees reported spending 100% of their work hours within the rail yard, while three (9%) reported spending fewer than 100% of their work hours within the rail yard. Of the interviewed employees, 28 (85%) reported operating an RCL device as part of their job.

Regarding exposures, 32 (97%) employees reported smelling diesel exhaust during their work in the rail yard at least some of the time. Two (6%) employees reported being exposed to diesel exhaust or fumes outside of work. Six (18%) employees reported that they were current smokers, while eight (24%) reported that they were

Table 3. Work characteristics of interviewed employees

Work Characteristic	No. (%) Employees n = 33
Job title	
Engineer	2 (6)
Conductor/trainman	31 (94)
Work location within rail yard	
Hump yard	6 (18)
Bowl yard	18 (55)
South yard	6 (18)
Other	3 (9)
Work shift	
First shift	13 (39)
Second shift	10 (30)
Third shift	10 (30)

former smokers. None of the employees reported working with any chemicals during their work in the rail yard.

One interviewed employee reported he had been diagnosed with prostate cancer, and one reported he has been diagnosed with chronic lymphocytic leukemia. The employee with prostate cancer was one of the 13 employees initially identified as having prostate cancer. No other employees reported a history of cancer (including leukemia or lymphoma).

Three (9%) employees reported ever having asthma, while 15 (45%) employees reported ever having hay fever or allergic rhinitis. One employee reported ever having both conditions. Of these 16 employees, six (38%) reported that their symptoms were worse while working in the rail yard or on the locomotives. None of the employees reported ever having emphysema or chronic bronchitis.

Symptoms reported while working in the rail yard or on the locomotives are shown in Table 4. These symptoms were attributed by the employees to various causes, including heat, seasonal allergies, and less often, diesel exhaust. Four (12%) employees reported experiencing none of the symptoms while working in the rail yard or on the locomotives.

Table 4. Symptoms reported by interviewed employees while working in the yard or on locomotives

Symptom Reported	No. (%) Employees n = 33
General symptoms	
Fatigue	25 (76)
Headache	19 (45)
Dizziness/lightheadedness	14 (42)
Loss of appetite	10 (30)
Facial flushing	8 (24)
Skin rash	2 (6)
Eyes, nose and throat symptoms	
Runny nose or congestion	15 (45)
Eye irritation	14 (42)
Sore throat/ irritation	7 (21)
Nosebleed	5 (15)
Respiratory symptoms	
Cough	9 (27)
Shortness of breath	7 (21)
Wheezing	3 (9)
Gastrointestinal symptoms	
Abdominal pain	4 (12)
Nausea	4 (12)
Vomiting	2 (6)

Elemental Carbon

Table 5 presents the elemental carbon personal air sampling results. The California OEL for diesel exhaust particles does not specify whether total or respirable elemental carbon sampling should be used [CDHS 2002], so we compared both the total and respirable elemental carbon concentrations to this OEL. All elemental carbon air concentrations were below the California OEL of 20 μg/m^3 [CDHS 2002] except for the personal air concentration measured on Switchman 5 who worked in the south yard and made a 2-hour "local industries" trip to a nearby coke plant on June 15, 2011, (20 μg/m^3). "Local industries" was the only process we sampled that involved riding on a locomotive outside the rail yard. All other air samples were collected from trainmen in the rail yard. Of these samples, the elemental carbon air concentration measured from Foreman 2 in the bowl yard on June 14, 2011, (18 μg/m^3) was outside the range of all the other measurements. After collection, we observed that the sample filter was much darker than all the other sample filters, suggesting that it had possibly been placed in or near the exhaust stream of a locomotive engine.

Table 6 displays the area air sampling results for elemental carbon. The area air concentrations of elemental carbon were on average lower and less variable than the personal air concentrations. A comparison of the total and respirable dust sampling results on the same employees (Table 5) suggested that 20% to 43% of the elemental carbon in the personal breathing zones was respirable. A comparison of the total and respirable dust sampling results from the same locations (Table 6) suggested that 38% to 61% of the elemental carbon in the air was respirable.

In addition to the elemental carbon, much of the organic carbon in air was respirable (data not shown). Overall, the respirable dust samples had fewer complex organic fractions based on the "thermograms" (evolution of carbon during analysis over different temperatures and atmospheres) than the total dust samples. High levels of some types of organic carbon particulate matter can contribute small amounts of elemental carbon through carbonization. Although combustion aerosol is known to be mainly submicrometer [Wichmann 2007], it is possible that larger agglomerates of elemental carbon were formed in the diesel exhaust of the locomotive engines. Size distribution measurements were not made near the engine exhaust to determine the particle size fraction.

The MDC and MQC for elemental carbon were calculated by dividing the respective analytical limits of detection and quantitation (mass units) by the average volume of air sampled (1.5 m^3). The MDC and MQC represent the smallest air concentrations that could have been detected (MDC) or quantified (MQC) on the basis of the volume of air sampled. Concentrations between the MDC and MQC are provided in Tables 5 and 6 in parentheses to indicate the greater level of uncertainty associated with these values.

Table 5. Personal air concentrations of elemental carbon measured during a work shift

Date	Process/ Location	Job Title	Type	Sample Time (min)	Elemental Carbon ($\mu g/m^3$)
6/14/2011	Bowl yard	Foreman 1	Total	328	1.8
			Respirable	328	0.77
		Foreman 2	Total	368	18
		Foreman 3	Total	290	4.3
			Respirable	290	0.85
		Switchman 1	Total	340	3.0
		Switchman 2	Total	358	3.7
		Switchman 3	Total	283	2.7
			Respirable	283	(0.54)
6/15/2011	Hump yard	Foreman 4	Total	442	3.2
	Local industries	Foreman 5	Total	454	6.6
			Respirable	454	1.7
		Engineer 1	Total	468	4.2
	Hump yard	Switchman 4	Total	325	1.9
			Respirable	325	0.77
	South yard/local industries	Switchman 5	Total	404	20
MDC					0.2
MQC					0.65
California OEL [CDHS 2002]					20

RESULTS
(CONTINUED)

Table 6. Area air concentrations of elemental carbon measured during a work shift

Date	Location	Type	Sample Time (min)	Elemental Carbon ($\mu g/m^3$)
6/14/2011	Next to the knuckle rack in the bowl yard	Total	208	1.8
		Respirable	208	(0.70)*
6/15/2011	Outside hump yard shack	Total	577	2.1
		Respirable	577	1.3
	100 yards north of the south tower	Total	446	2.6
		Respirable	446	1.1
MDC				0.2
MQC				0.65

*Volume of air collected (0.8 m³) was less than the volume of air used to calculate the MDC and MQC (1.5 m³).

Oxides of Nitrogen, Sulfur, and Carbon

Work-shift average personal air concentrations of NO ranged from ND to 0.001 ppm, and work-shift average personal air concentrations of NO_2 ranged from ND to 0.003 ppm. These averages are well below applicable work-shift OELs (Table 7). Peak instantaneous measurements of NO_2 (< 0.7 ppm) were well below applicable short-term exposure limits and ceiling limits (Table 7). The SO_2 and CO meters did not log data as intended. Therefore, we are unable to present the results of those measurements. However, the CO meter worn by Switchman 5 on June 15, 2011, alarmed during a trip to a nearby coke plant, indicating the meter was exposed to a CO concentration >35 ppm. During this trip the switchman described smelling something that burned his nose and stung his tongue, two symptoms associated with exposure to acids. Because CO meters have known cross sensitivities with some acids, following our evaluation, an industrial hygienist from the railroad company conducted more CO air sampling to identify the cause of the alarm. In this subsequent sampling this industrial hygienist discovered that the CO meter alarmed when it was near the locomotive's battery compartment. Upon closer inspection, the industrial hygienist determined that the locomotive battery was leaking acid. This explains both why the NIOSH CO meter alarmed and the switchman's temporary symptoms. To our knowledge, none of the other SO_2 or CO meters alarmed. Although these meters did not log data, we have no reason to believe that they measured levels exceeding the applicable OELs (Table 7).

Table 7. Exposure limits (ppm) for the oxides of nitrogen, sulfur, and carbon that were measured

Agency or Association	Type of OEL	NO	NO_2	SO_2	CO
NIOSH REL*	Work shift OEL	25	NA	2	35
	STEL	NA	1	5	200
OSHA PEL*	Work shift OEL	25	NA	5	50
	Ceiling limit	NA	5	NA	NA
ACGIH TLV[†]	Work shift OEL	25	3	NA	25
	STEL	NA	5	0.25	NA

*[NIOSH 2010]
[†][ACGIH 2011]

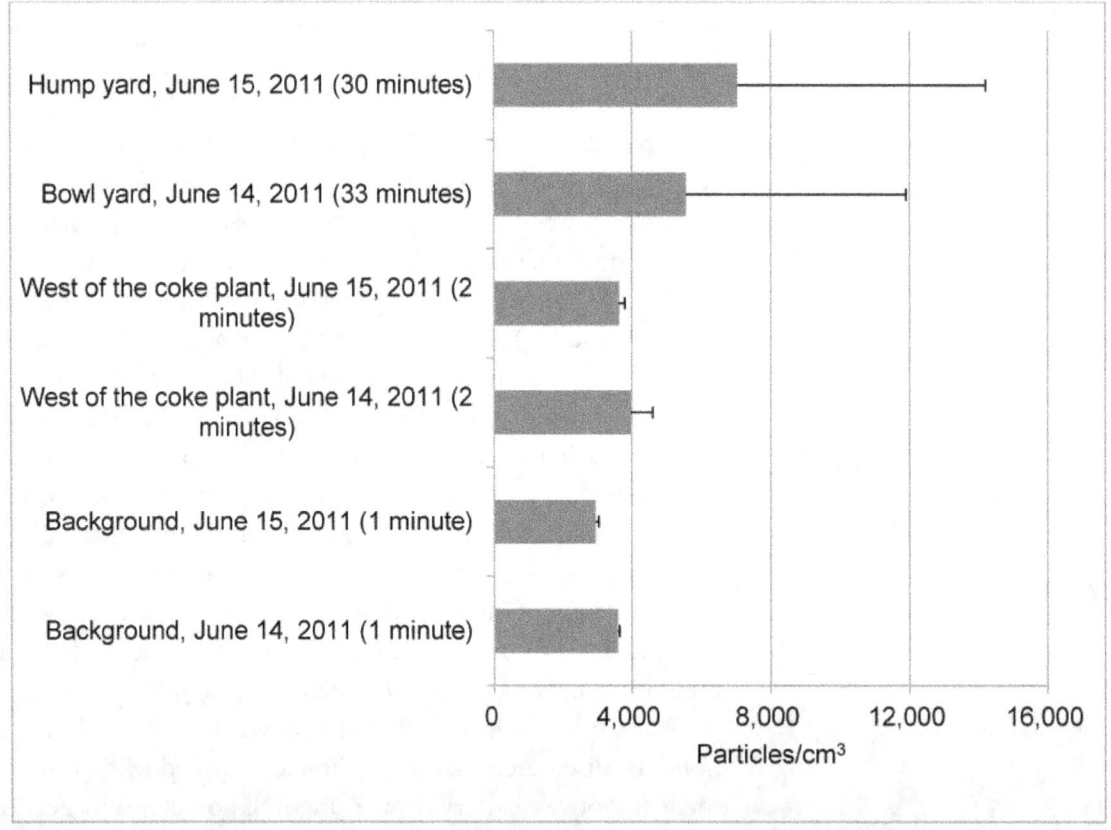

Figure 2. Average fine particle count concentrations and standard deviations (error bars) measured at or near the rail yard.

Fine Particles

Figure 2 summarizes the fine particle measurements collected at or near the rail yard. On average, the concentration of airborne particles measured in the rail yard (6,700 particles/cm^3) was 1 9 times higher than those measured outside the rail yard (3,500 particles/cm^3). Background measurements were collected in a residential area about 1 mile northeast of the rail yard near a horse farm. The coke plant east of the rail yard did not appear to contribute to the fine particles in the rail yard air. According to the National Climatic Data Center [http://www.ncdc noaa.gov], the wind was predominately out of the north on June 14, 2011, (average 4 miles per hour) and out of the west on June 15, 2011, (average 5.4 miles per hour). Thus, the rail yard was upwind of the coke plant. The sample times and variability for the measurements collected at the rail yard were substantially higher than for the other measurements.

Radio Frequency

The applicable OELs for the operating frequencies of the RCL devices (450–470 MHz) and two-way radios (136–174 MHz) are provided in Table 8. These OELs are primarily intended to prevent adverse heating of biological tissue. We had a difficult time measuring the power density levels from the RCL devices because they transmitted on shared time slots, and the exposures were brief and intermittent. However, when we did measure the transmission, the maximum power density levels were <10% of the most conservative OEL (1.1 mW/cm^2 [ICNIRP 1998]). It is important to note that ceiling limits for power density levels do not exist. To comply with the OELs for 450–470 MHz, measurements should be collected and averaged over a 6-minute period. Doing so in this situation would inevitably lead to even lower levels than the maximum levels we measured. For example, the average levels during 1-minute sampling periods were near zero mW/cm^2.

The maximum power density level during a two-way radio transmission was five times higher than the most conservative OEL (0.2 mW/cm^2 [ICNIRP 1998]). However, to comply with this OEL, measurements should be collected and averaged over a 30-minute period (or 6-minute period for the other OELs). Because the two-way radios were typically operated continuously for less than 10 seconds at a time, averaging over 30 minutes or even 6 minutes would inevitably lead to much lower levels. For example, the average level during a 1-minute sampling period was near zero mW/cm^2.

Table 8. OELs (6 minute averages unless otherwise noted) for radio frequency power density levels (mW/cm^2)

Frequency (MHz)	ICNIRP [ICNIRP 1998]	FCC [FCC 1999]	IEEE [IEEE 2005]	ACGIH [ACGIH 2011]
450–470	1.1	1.5	1.5	1.5
136–174	0.2*	1	1	1

*Averaged over 30 minutes

Work Practice Observations

During our visit, we observed good adherence among employees to measures that reduce the potential for heat stress, including frequent hydration, use of hats, and going into the shade when possible. However, we observed inconsistent and suboptimal use of hearing protection in the south, hump, and bowl yards. These observations were verified by many employees who reported noncompliance with hearing protection during the interviews. Many of these employees reported that they were unable to hear necessary communication through their radios when wearing hearing protection. We also learned from employer representatives that the railroad company conducted audiometric tests on rail yard employees every 3 years.

DISCUSSION

Cancer Cluster Investigation

Background on Cancer Clusters

Cancers often appear to occur in clusters, which are defined as "unusual aggregations, real or perceived, of health events that are grouped together in time and space" [CDC 1990]. A cluster also occurs when the same type of cancers are found among workers of a different age or sex group than is usual. These cancer cases may have a common cause or may be the coincidental occurrence of unrelated causes. The number of cases of all types of cancer may seem high, particularly among the small group of people who have something in common with the cases, such as working in the same building. However, many people fail to consider how common cancer is in this country, especially in an aging workforce.

Diseases often are not distributed randomly in the population, and clusters of disease may arise by chance alone [Metz 1997]. In many workplaces, the number of cases is small. This makes it difficult for us to detect whether the cases have a common cause, especially in the absence of apparent cancer-causing exposures. It is common for the borders of the perceived cluster to be drawn around where the cases of cancer are located, instead of defining the population and geographic area first. This often leads to the inaccurate belief that the rate of cancer is high.

Our Methodology in Cancer Cluster Investigations

In conducting an investigation of a perceived excess of cancer occurring among employees of the same workplace, we begin by gathering data on those employees diagnosed with cancer. When cancer in a workplace is described, learning whether the type of cancer is a primary cancer or a metastasis (spread of the primary cancer into other organs) is important. Only primary cancers are used to investigate a cancer cluster. To assess whether the cancers among employees could be related to occupational exposures, we consider the number of cancer cases, the types of cancer, the likelihood of exposure to potential cancer-causing agents, and the timing of the diagnosis of cancer in relation to the exposure. These issues are discussed below as they relate to the request.

Do transportation department employees at the rail yard have more cancer than people who do not work at the rail yard?

When several cases of cancer occur in a workplace, they may be part of a true cluster when the number is greater than we expect compared to other groups of people similar in age, sex, and race. Disease or tumor rates, however, are highly variable in small populations and rarely match the overall rate for a larger area, such as the state, so that for any given time period some populations have rates above the overall rate and others have rates below the overall rate. So, even when a higher rate occurs, this may be completely consistent with the expected random variability. In addition, calculations like this make many assumptions that may not be appropriate for every workplace. Comparing rates without adjusting for age, sex, or other population characteristics assumes that such characteristics are the same in the workplace as in the larger population, which may not be true.

Eight current and former transportation department employees at the rail yard were identified as having been diagnosed with prostate cancer from 1999 to present. In the United States, one in six men will develop prostate cancer over the course of his lifetime, and prostate cancer is the most frequently diagnosed cancer in men. Because the total number of transportation department employees over this 12 year period was quite large, this was not an unusual number of cases.

Is exposure to a specific chemical or physical agent known or suspected of causing cancer occurring?

The relationship between some agents and certain cancers has been well established. For other agents and cancers, including prostate cancer, there is a suspicion, but the evidence is not definitive. When a known or suspected cancer-causing agent is present and the types of cancer occurring have been linked with these exposures in other settings, we are more likely to make the connection between cancer and a workplace exposure.

No occupational or environmental risk factors for prostate cancer are known, and rail transport workers have not consistently been shown to have a statistically significant excess of diagnosed prostate cancer [Aronson et al. 1996; Krstev et al. 1998a; Krstev et al. 1998b]. Exposure to certain substances, such as polycyclic aromatic hydrocarbons, pesticides, and cadmium have been suspected to increase the risk for prostate cancer, but study results conflict [Verougstraete et al. 2003; Boers et al. 2005; Sahmoun et al. 2005; Van Maele-Fabry et al. 2006; Huff et al. 2007; Mink et al. 2008]. In addition, a systematic review and meta-analysis of eight studies did not conclude that occupational exposure to whole-body vibration was a risk factor for prostate cancer [Young et al. 2009].

The only well-established risk factors for prostate cancer are age $\geq$ 50 years, African-American race, and having a family history of the disease [American Cancer Society 2011]. All eight interviewed employees who were diagnosed with prostate cancer had at least one known risk factor for prostate cancer.

Has enough time passed since exposure began?

The latency period is the time between first exposure to a cancer-causing agent and clinical recognition of the disease. Latency periods vary by cancer type but are usually 15–20 years or longer and are usually a minimum of 10–12 years [Rugo 2004]. For example, it can take up to 30 years after exposure to asbestos for mesothelioma to develop. Because of this, past exposures are more relevant than current exposures as potential causes of cancers occurring in workers today. However, with the absence of documented workplace exposures at the rail yard, consideration of latency was not a factor in this HHE.

Evaluation of Exposures at the Rail Yard

Most (88%) employees reported experiencing at least one health symptom during their work at the rail yard or on the locomotives. These symptoms included general ear, nose, and throat; respiratory; and gastrointestinal symptoms. These symptoms were attributed by the employees to various causes, including heat, seasonal allergies, and less often, diesel exhaust. It is difficult to determine a cause of the reported symptoms because they can have multiple causes and are common in the general population.

Because diesel exhaust is a potential lung carcinogen [NIOSH 1988; IARC 1989], it is advisable to maintain occupational exposures as low as feasible. Most of the personal air concentrations of elemental carbon we measured were less than half of the California OEL. However, two personal concentrations were near or at the California OEL. Both of these measurements were collected with the total dust sampler. On the basis of our comparison of the respirable and total elemental carbon area air concentrations, the total dust sample results may overestimate the actual levels of elemental carbon attributable to diesel exhaust due to the presence of other carbonaceous particulate (e.g., coal dust). Alternatively, it is possible that agglomerated particles larger than the cyclone cut point (4.2 μm) were present in the locomotive diesel exhaust emissions. Additional sampling is necessary to determine whether this is the case. In addition, the air sample collected from Foreman 2 in the bowl yard was possibly placed in the exhaust stream of a diesel engine, and other sources of elemental carbon at the coke plant (i.e., factory emissions and other diesel engines) may have contributed to the higher exposure for Switchman 5.

If the wind had been blowing out of the east, then the coke plant could have contributed to the airborne elemental carbon levels measured for the transportation department employees at the rail yard. However, the wind was blowing from the north or west during our evaluation and the direct-reading fine particle measurements collected just west of the coke plant were near background levels. According to our fine particle measurements, the locomotive engines were the primary source of diesel exhaust at the rail yard. However, it is possible that coke plant emissions may have deposited in the rail yard (at some point in the past) and were resuspended in the air during our sample collection.

Diesel exhaust exposures at the rail yard are likely to vary over time because of differences in environmental conditions (temperature, humidity, wind speed, wind direction, etc.), workplace conditions (number of locomotives, age of locomotives, etc.), and human factors (time spent outdoors, time spent near idling engines, riding in locomotives with open windows, etc.). Consequently, our sampling results may not be representative of an employee's exposure throughout the year. However, the personal air concentrations of elemental carbon we measured are comparable to those in the railroad company's sampling records for other rail yards (geometric mean 1.6 µg/m^3 with an estimated 95th percentile of 15 µg/m^3). A review paper [Pronk et al. 2009] summarizing diesel exhaust measurements in various industries reported a geometric mean personal concentration of elemental carbon for non-operating train crew of 6 µg/m^3 (inhalable particles). Inhalable particles are more appropriately compared to our total elemental carbon results. The geometric mean personal concentration of total elemental carbon that we measured was 4.5 µg/m^3.

This same review paper [Pronk et al. 2009] also reported average personal air concentrations of NO (1.1 ppm), NO_2 (0.3 ppm), and CO (4.5 ppm) for non-operating train crew. We measured lower work-shift average personal air concentrations of NO (<0.002 ppm) and NO_2 (<0.004 ppm). The personal air concentrations of CO were likely below or comparable to the measurements reported in the review paper, but we cannot be certain because the meters did not log data. Because the diesel fuel used in locomotives at the rail yard had ultra-low sulfur content [BP 2010], it is unlikely that the SO_2 concentrations from the locomotive diesel exhaust would exceed applicable OELs.

Many of the transportation department employees operated RCL devices and two-way radios during a portion of the work day and could receive radio frequency exposures from both devices. The RCL devices and two-way radios were low power and approved for

DISCUSSION (CONTINUED)

use by the FCC. On the basis of our power density measurements and the transmission frequency of the devices, employees are unlikely to be overexposed to radio frequencies. The potential for overexposure does exist with the two-way radios but only if they were operated continuously for several minutes at a time. This duration of use would require further evaluation of radio frequency exposures. However, we did not observe this duration of use among the employees we monitored. Typically, the two-way radios were operated for < 10 seconds at a time.

CONCLUSIONS

The number of prostate cancer cases identified among current and former employees at the rail yard did not appear to be unusual. We do not believe that cancer reported among workers were the result of working at the rail yard. While most interviewed employees reported experiencing at least one health symptom while working, the nonspecific symptoms can be attributed to various etiologies including heat, underlying seasonal allergies, and asthma. The components of diesel exhaust that we measured in air were generally low (below applicable OELs). Other sources of elemental carbon may have contributed to one overexposure, but this requires further evaluation. Because diesel exhaust is a potential lung carcinogen [NIOSH 1988, IARC 1989,], it is advisable to maintain occupational exposures as low as feasible. Our measurements of power density levels suggest that the transportation department employees were unlikely to be overexposed to radio frequencies.

RECOMMENDATIONS

On the basis of our findings, we recommend the actions listed below to create a more healthful workplace. We encourage the rail yard to use a labor-management health and safety committee or working group to discuss the recommendations in this report and develop an action plan. Those involved in the work can best set priorities and assess the feasibility of our recommendations for the specific situation at the rail yard.

1. Conduct air sampling for elemental carbon focusing on the positions with the highest personal air concentrations. It is especially important to determine if the trip to the coke plant was a contributing factor to the overexposure for Switchman 5 and if so, what the relative contribution was from the locomotive's engine. This information can then be used to select the best control measures to minimize exposures.

2. Provide more detailed education on the RCL devices during the initial and refresher training for operators. Include explanations on the differences between ionizing and non-ionizing radiation, the radio frequencies and power densities at which the RCL devices and two-way radios operate, and the potential health effects from these devices.

3. Encourage employees to learn more about known cancer risk factors, particularly those for prostate cancer, and the measures they can take to reduce exposure to those risk factors within their control. Modifiable personal risk factors that are associated with certain types of cancer include tobacco use, high alcohol consumption, a diet low in fruits and vegetables, physical inactivity, and obesity. Employees should also discuss available cancer screening programs according to age, sex, or family history with their primary care physicians.

   More general information on cancer can be found on the American Cancer Society website at http://www.cancer.org and the National Cancer Institute website at http://www.cancer.gov. In addition, more information about occupational cancer and cancer cluster evaluations can be found on the NIOSH website at http://www.cdc.gov/niosh/topics/cancer.

4. Encourage employees to evaluate the quality of the health information that they find on the Internet. It is important to ensure that health information is reliable, up-to-date, and unbiased. The National Library of Medicine and the National Institutes of Health offer guidelines for evaluating the quality of health information on the Internet on their website at http://www.nlm.nih.gov/medlineplus/evaluatinghealthinformation.html.

5. Ensure that employees know to whom they should report any possible work-related health problems. Encourage employees to notify appropriate management representatives in a timely manner.

RECOMMENDATIONS (CONTINUED)

6. Conduct and analyze annual audiometric tests on rail yard employees. Although the Federal Railroad Administration only requires audiometric testing every 3 years, NIOSH recommends audiometric testing yearly [NIOSH 1998]. Annual audiometric testing is more likely to identify hearing loss early, allowing controls to be implemented to prevent further hearing loss.

7. Make the push-in style of earplugs more accessible to all employees. Because the policy at the rail yard is to require hearing protection within 100 feet of an operating locomotive, earplugs are likely to be worn intermittently. The push-in style of earplugs is easier to insert in the ear canal than moldable foam earplugs. This may increase the use of earplugs at the rail yard. As an alternative, consider using communication earmuffs to facilitate radio communications while providing hearing protection. It is important to select hearing protection that does not over-attenuate noise based on measured noise levels.

8. Install signs near the hump yard to notify employees that they are entering an area where hearing protection is required. This will remind employees to wear earplugs in this high noise area.

REFERENCES

ACGIH [2006]. Radiofrequency and microwave radiation In: Documentation of the threshold limit values and biological exposure indices. Cincinnati, OH: American Conference of Governmental Industrial Hygienists.

ACGIH [2011]. Threshold limit values for chemical substances and physical agents and biological exposure indices. Cincinnati, OH: American Conference of Governmental Industrial Hygienists.

American Cancer Society [2011]. Cancer Facts & Figures 2011. Atlanta, Georgia: American Cancer Society.

ANSI [2002]. Mechanical vibration and shock: evaluation of human exposure to whole-body vibration - Part 1: general requirements. American National Standards Institute, Inc. ANSI S3.18-2002.

Aronson KJ, Siemiatycki J, Dewar R, Gerin M [1996]. Occupational risk factors for prostate cancer: results from a case-control study in Montréal, Québec, Canada. Am J Epidemiol 143(4):363–373.

Boers D, Zeegers MPA, Swaen GM, Kant I, van den Brandt PA [2005]. The influence of occupational exposure to pesticides, polycyclic aromatic hydrocarbons, diesel exhaust, metal dust, metal fumes, and mineral oil on prostate cancer: a prospective cohort study. Occup Environ Med 62(8):531–537.

BP [2010]. Material safety data sheet: diesel fuel no. 2. Naperville, Illinois: British Petroleum (BP). MSDS #11155.

Canada Center for Occupational Health and Safety [2011]. Vibration: health effects. [http://www.ccohs.ca/oshanswers/phys_agents/vibration/vibration_effects.html]. Date accessed: October 2011.

CDC (Centers for Disease Control) [1990]. Guidelines for investigating clusters of health events. MMWR 39(11).

CDHS [2002]. Health hazard advisory: diesel engine exhaust. Oakland, California: Hazard Evaluation System and Information Service, California Department of Health Services (CDHS), Occupational Health Branch. [http://www.cdph.ca.gov/programs/hesis/Documents/diesel.pdf]. Date accessed: October 2011.

EPA [2002]. Health assessment document for diesel engine exhaust. Washington, DC: National Center for Environmental Assessment, Office of Transportation and Air Quality, U.S. Environmental Protection Agency (EPA) Publication No. EPA/600/8-90/057F.

FCC [1999]. Questions and answers about biological effects and potential hazards of radiofrequency electromagnetic fields. By Cleveland RF, Ulcek JL. Washington D.C.: U.S. Federal Communications Commission (FCC), OET bulletin 56, 4th ed.

Huff J, Lunn RM, Waalkes MP, Tomatis L, Infante PF [2007]. Cadmium-induced cancers in animals and in humans. Int J Occup Environ Health 13(2):202–212.

REFERENCES
(CONTINUED)

IARC [1989]. IARC monographs on the evaluation of carcinogenic risks to humans: diesel and engine exhausts and some nitroarenes. Vol 46. Lyon, France: International Agency for Research on Cancer (IARC).

ICNIRP [1998]. Guidelines for limiting exposure to time-varying electric, magnetic, and electromagnetic fields (up to 300 GHz). Oberschleissheim, Germany: International Commission on Non-Ionizing Radiation Protection (ICNIRP).

IEEE [2005]. IEEE standard for safety levels with respect to human exposure to radio frequency electromagnetic fields, 3 kHz to 300 GHz. New York: Institute of Electrical and Electronics Engineers (IEEE). Standard C95.1-2005.

Krstev S, Baris D, Stewart P, Dosemeci M, Swanson GM, Greenberg RS, Schoenberg JB, Schwartz AG, Liff JM, Hayes RB [1998a]. Occupational risk factors and prostate cancer in U.S. blacks and whites. Am J Ind Med 34(5):421–430.

Krstev S, Baris D, Stewart PA, Hayes RB, Blair A, Dosemeci M [1998b]. Risk for prostate cancer by occupation and industry: a 24-state death certificate study. Am J Ind Med 34(5):413–420.

Metz LM, McGuinness S [1997]. Responding to reported clusters of common diseases: the case of multiple sclerosis. Can J Public Health 99(4):277–279.

Mink PJ, Adami H-O, Trichopoulos D, Britton NL, Mandel JS [2008]. Pesticides and prostate cancer: a review of epidemiologic studies with specific agricultural exposure information. Europ J Cancer Prev 17(2):97–110.

NIOSH [1988]. Current intelligence bulletin 50: Carcinogenic effects of exposure to diesel exhaust. Cincinnati, OH: U.S. Department of Health and Human Services, Public Health Service, Centers for Disease Control and Prevention, National Institute for Occupational Safety and Health, DHHS (NIOSH) Publication No. 88-116.

NIOSH [1998]. Criteria for a recommended standard: Occupational noise exposure, revised criteria 1998. Cincinnati, OH: U.S. Department of Health and Human Services, Public Health Service, Centers for Disease Control and Prevention, National Institute for Occupational Safety and Health, DHHS (NIOSH) Publication No. 98-126. [http://www.cdc.gov/niosh/docs/98-126/]. Date accessed: October 2011.

NIOSH [2010]. NIOSH pocket guide to chemical hazards. Cincinnati, OH: U.S. Department of Health and Human Services, Centers for Disease Control and Prevention, National Institute for Occupational Safety and Health, DHHS (NIOSH) Publication No. 2010-168c. [http://www.cdc.gov/niosh/npg/]. Date accessed: October 2011.

NIOSH [2011]. NIOSH manual of analytical methods. 4th ed. Schlecht PC, O'Connor PF, eds. Cincinnati, OH: U.S. Department of Health and Human Services, Centers for Disease Control and Prevention, National Institute for Occupational Safety and Health, DHHS (NIOSH) Publication No. 94-113 (August 1994); 1st Supplement Publication 96-135, 2nd Supplement Publication 98-119, 3rd Supplement Publication 2003-154. [http://www.cdc.gov/niosh/docs/2003-154/]. Date accessed: October 2011.

OSHA [1988]. Hazard information bulletin on potential carcinogenicity of diesel exhaust. Washington, DC; U.S. Department of Labor, Occupational Safety and Health Administration. OSHA Bulletin 19881130.

Pronk A, Coble J, Stewart PA [2009]. Occupational exposure to diesel engine exhaust: a literature review. J Expo Sci Environ Epidemiol 19(5):443–457.

Rugo H [2004]. Occupational cancer. In: LaDou J, ed. Current occupational and environmental medicine. New York: McGraw Hill Companies, Inc., pp. 229–267.

Sahmoun AE, Case LD, Jackson SA, Schwartz GG [2005]. Cadmium and prostate cancer: a critical epidemiologic analysis. Cancer Invest 23(3):256–263.

REFERENCES (CONTINUED)

Van Maele-Fabry G, Libotte V, Willems J, Lison D [2006]. Review and meta-analysis of risk estimates for prostate cancer in pesticide manufacturing workers. Cancer Causes Control 17(4):353–373.

Verougstraete V, Lison D, Hotz P [2003]. Cadmium, lung and prostate cancer: a systematic review of recent epidemiological data. J Toxicol Environ Health 6(3):227–255.

Wichmann HE [2007]. Diesel exhaust particles. Inhal Toxicol 19 Suppl 1:241–244.

Young E, Kreiger N, Purdham J, Sass-Kortsak A [2009]. Prostate cancer and driving occupations: could whole body vibration play a role? Int Arch Occup Environ Health 82(5):551–556.

In evaluating the hazards posed by workplace exposures, NIOSH investigators use both mandatory (legally enforceable) and recommended OELs for chemical, physical, and biological agents as a guide for making recommendations. OELs have been developed by federal agencies and safety and health organizations to prevent the occurrence of adverse health effects from workplace exposures. Generally, OELs suggest levels of exposure that most employees may be exposed to for up to 10 hours per day, 40 hours per week, for a working lifetime, without experiencing adverse health effects. However, not all employees will be protected from adverse health effects even if their exposures are maintained below these levels. A small percentage may experience adverse health effects because of individual susceptibility, a preexisting medical condition, and/or a hypersensitivity (allergy). In addition, some hazardous substances may act in combination with other workplace exposures, the general environment, or with medications or personal habits of the employee to produce adverse health effects even if the occupational exposures are controlled at the level set by the exposure limit. Also, some substances can be absorbed by direct contact with the skin and mucous membranes in addition to being inhaled, which contributes to the individual's overall exposure.

Most OELs are expressed as a TWA exposure. A TWA refers to the average exposure during a normal 8- to 10-hour workday. Some chemical substances and physical agents have recommended STEL or ceiling values where adverse health effects are caused by exposures over a short period. Unless otherwise noted, the STEL is a 15-minute TWA exposure that should not be exceeded at any time during a workday, and the ceiling limit is an exposure that should not be exceeded at any time.

In the United States, OELs have been established by federal agencies, professional organizations, state and local governments, and other entities. Some OELs are legally enforceable limits, while others are recommendations. The U.S. Department of Labor OSHA PELs (29 CFR 1910 [general industry]; 29 CFR 1926 [construction industry]; and 29 CFR 1917 [maritime industry]) are legal limits enforceable in workplaces covered under the Occupational Safety and Health Act of 1970. NIOSH RELs are recommendations based on a critical review of the scientific and technical information available on a given hazard and the adequacy of methods to identify and control the hazard. NIOSH RELs can be found in the NIOSH Pocket Guide to Chemical Hazards [NIOSH 2010]. NIOSH also recommends different types of risk management practices (e.g., engineering controls, safe work practices, employee education/ training, personal protective equipment, and exposure and medical monitoring) to minimize the risk of exposure and adverse health effects from these hazards. Other OELs that are commonly used and cited in the United States include the TLVs recommended by ACGIH, a professional organization, and the WEELs recommended by the American Industrial Hygiene Association, another professional organization. The TLVs and WEELs are developed by committee members of these associations from a review of the published, peer-reviewed literature. They are not consensus standards. ACGIH TLVs are considered voluntary exposure guidelines for use by industrial hygienists and others trained in this discipline "to assist in the control of health hazards" [ACGIH 2011]. WEELs have been established for some chemicals "when no other legal or authoritative limits exist" [AIHA 2011].

Outside the United States, OELs have been established by various agencies and organizations and include both legal and recommended limits. The Institut für Arbeitsschutz der Deutschen Gesetzlichen Unfallversicherung (IFA, Institute for Occupational Safety and Health of the German Social Accident

APPENDIX: OCCUPATIONAL EXPOSURE LIMITS AND HEALTH EFFECTS (CONTINUED)

Insurance) maintains a database of international OELs from European Union member states, Canada (Québec), Japan, Switzerland, and the United States. The database, available at http://www.dguv.de/ifa/en/gestis/limit_values/index.jsp, contains international limits for over 1,500 hazardous substances and is updated periodically.

Employers should understand that not all hazardous chemicals have specific OSHA PELs, and for some agents the legally enforceable and recommended limits may not reflect current health-based information. However, an employer is still required by OSHA to protect its employees from hazards even in the absence of a specific OSHA PEL. OSHA requires an employer to furnish employees a place of employment free from recognized hazards that cause or are likely to cause death or serious physical harm [Occupational Safety and Health Act of 1970 (Public Law 91–596, sec. 5(a)(1))]. Thus, NIOSH investigators encourage employers to make use of other OELs when making risk assessments and risk management decisions to best protect the health of their employees. NIOSH investigators also encourage the use of the traditional hierarchy of controls approach to eliminate or minimize identified workplace hazards. This includes, in order of preference, the use of (1) substitution or elimination of the hazardous agent, (2) engineering controls (e.g., local exhaust ventilation, process enclosure, dilution ventilation), (3) administrative controls (e.g., limiting time of exposure, employee training, work practice changes, medical surveillance), and (4) personal protective equipment (e.g., respiratory protection, gloves, eye protection, hearing protection). Control banding, a qualitative risk assessment and risk management tool, is a complementary approach to protecting employee health that focuses resources on exposure controls by describing how a risk needs to be managed. Information on control banding is available at http://www.cdc.gov/niosh/topics/ctrlbanding/. This approach can be applied in situations where OELs have not been established or can be used to supplement the OELs, when available.

The following sections provide more information about the OELs and health effects pertaining to diesel exhaust and radio frequencies.

Diesel Exhaust

Diesel exhaust is a complex mixture of thousands of gases and fine particles (commonly known as soot) that contains more than 40 potentially toxic compounds [EPA 2002]. The particulate fraction of diesel exhaust is composed of microscopic cores of elemental carbon onto which are adsorbed thousands of substances [NIOSH 1988; OSHA 1988]. The adsorbed material contributes 15% to 65% of the total particulate mass and includes compounds such as polycyclic aromatic hydrocarbons, many of which are possibly carcinogenic [NIOSH 1988; OSHA 1988; ARB 1998]. Because of their small size (< 2.5 μm in aerodynamic diameter) [Wichmann 2007], diesel exhaust particles can be inhaled deeply into the lungs where they are more difficult to clear [Hinds 1999]. Some of the main toxic gases in diesel exhaust are oxides of nitrogen, sulfur, and carbon [NIOSH 1988; OSHA 1988].

Acute health effects of diesel exhaust exposure include irritation of the eyes, nose, throat, and lungs, and it can cause cough, headache, lightheadedness, and nausea [Reger and Hancock 1980; Gamble et al.

1987; Sydbom et al. 2001]. Exposure to diesel exhaust can also cause inflammation in the lungs, which may aggravate chronic respiratory symptoms and asthma. Chronic exposures are associated with cough, increased sputum production, and lung function changes [Ulfvarson and Alexandersson 1990; Sydbom et al. 2001]. Whether a person experiences these acute or chronic health effects depends on the magnitude of their exposures and on individual susceptibility.

Diesel exhaust is considered a probable human carcinogen [IARC 1989]. On the basis of the results of laboratory animal and human epidemiology studies, NIOSH considers whole diesel exhaust emissions a potential occupational carcinogen [NIOSH 1988]. Human epidemiology studies suggest an association between occupational exposure to whole diesel exhaust emissions and lung cancer [NIOSH 1988; ARB 1998; Garshick et. al 2004], while studies of rats and mice exposed to whole diesel exhaust, and especially to the particulate portion, confirm an association with lung tumors [NIOSH 1988; OSHA 1988; ARB 1998]. NIOSH has stated that "excess cancer risk for workers exposed to diesel exhaust has not yet been quantified, but the probability of developing cancer should be reduced by minimizing exposure" [NIOSH 1988].

Federally mandated OELs exist for NO, NO_2, SO_2, and CO (Table 7); however, at the present time, no federally mandated OELs exist for diesel exhaust. On the basis of the risk assessment performed by the California Environmental Protection Agency, Office of Environmental Health Hazard Assessment, exposure to 20 μg/m³ of diesel exhaust particles over a working lifetime would create an excess lung cancer risk of one in a thousand. This level is often considered an acceptable workplace risk and was used as the basis of the California OEL [CDHS 2002].

Radio Frequency

The OELs listed in Table 8 are ICNIRP reference levels for occupational exposures [ICNIRP 1998], IEEE maximum permissible exposures for the upper tier (people in controlled environments) [IEEE 2005], ACGIH TLVs [ACGIH 2011], and FCC limits for occupational/controlled exposure [FCC 1999] for radio frequencies.

The ICNIRP reference levels are based on short-term, immediate health effects such as stimulation of peripheral nerves and muscles, shocks and burns caused by touching conducting objects, and elevated tissue temperatures resulting from absorption of energy [ICNIRP 1998]. The FCC limits are intended to prevent similar health effects [FCC 1999]. The IEEE maximum permissible exposures specifically for 100 kHz to 300 GHz are intended to protect against adverse heating of biological tissues [IEEE 2005]. The ACGIH TLVs are based upon the belief that the primary adverse physiological effects of electromagnetic energy in this wavelength and frequency region are thermal [ACGIH 2006]. Two areas of the body, the eyes and the testes, are known to be particularly vulnerable to heating by radio frequency energy because of the relative lack of available blood flow to dissipate the excessive heat load. Intense radio frequency exposures to the eyes of animals have been shown to cause cataracts. Intense radio frequency exposures to the testes of animals have been shown to cause temporary sterility [FCC 1999].

References

ACGIH [2006]. Radiofrequency and microwave radiation In: Documentation of the threshold limit values and biological exposure indices. Cincinnati, OH: American Conference of Governmental Industrial Hygienists.

ACGIH [2011]. Threshold limit values for chemical substances and physical agents and biological exposure indices. Cincinnati, OH: American Conference of Governmental Industrial Hygienists.

AIHA [2011]. AIHA 2011 Emergency response planning guidelines (ERPG) & workplace environmental exposure levels (WEEL) handbook. Fairfax, VA: American Industrial Hygiene Association.

ARB [1998]. The report on diesel exhaust. Sacramento, California: California Environmental Protection Agency, California Air Resources Board (ARB). April 22, 1998.

CDHS [2002]. Health hazard advisory: diesel engine exhaust. Oakland, California: Hazard Evaluation System and Information Service, California Department of Health Services (CDHS), Occupational Health Branch. [http://www.cdph.ca.gov/programs/hesis/Documents/diesel.pdf]. Date accessed: October 2011.

CFR. Code of Federal Regulations. Washington, DC: U.S. Government Printing Office, Office of the Federal Register.

EPA [2002]. Health assessment document for diesel engine exhaust. Washington, DC: National Center for Environmental Assessment, Office of Transportation and Air Quality, U.S. Environmental Protection Agency (EPA) Publication No. EPA/600/8-90/057F.

FCC [1999]. Questions and answers about biological effects and potential hazards of radiofrequency electromagnetic fields. By Cleveland RF, Ulcek JL. Washington D.C.: U.S. Federal Communications Commission (FCC), OET bulletin 56, 4th ed.

Gamble J, Jones W, Mishall S [1987]. Epidemiological-environmental study of diesel bus garage workers: acute effects of NO_2 and respirable particulate on the respiratory system. Environ Res 42(1):201–214.

Garshick E, Laden F, Hart JE, Rosner B, Smith TJ, Dockery D, Speizer FE [2004]. Lung cancer in railroad workers exposed to diesel exhaust. Environ Health Perspect 112(15):1539–1543.

Hinds WC [1999]. Respiratory deposition. In: Aerosol technology: properties, behavior, and measurement of airborne particles. New York: John Wiley & Sons, Inc.

IARC [1989]. IARC monographs on the evaluation of carcinogenic risks to humans: diesel and engine exhausts and some nitroarenes. Vol 46. Lyon, France: International Agency for Research on Cancer.

ICNIRP [1998]. Guidelines for limiting exposure to time-varying electric, magnetic, and electromagnetic fields (up to 300 GHz). Oberschleissheim, Germany: International Commission on Non-Ionizing Radiation Protection.

IEEE [2005]. IEEE standard for safety levels with respect to human exposure to radio frequency electromagnetic fields, 3 kHz to 300 GHz. New York: Institute of Electrical and Electronics Engineers. Standard C95.1-2005.

NIOSH [1988]. Current intelligence bulletin 50: Carcinogenic effects of exposure to diesel exhaust. Cincinnati, OH: U.S. Department of Health and Human Services, Public Health Service, Centers for Disease Control and Prevention, National Institute for Occupational Safety and Health, DHHS (NIOSH) Publication No. 88-116.

NIOSH [2010]. NIOSH pocket guide to chemical hazards. Cincinnati, OH: U.S. Department of Health and Human Services, Centers for Disease Control and Prevention, National Institute for Occupational Safety and Health, DHHS (NIOSH) Publication No. 2010-168c. [http://www.cdc.gov/niosh/npg]. Date accessed: October 2011.

OSHA [1988]. Hazard information bulletin on potential carcinogenicity of diesel exhaust. Washington, DC; U.S. Department of Labor, Occupational Safety and Health Administration. OSHA Bulletin 19881130.

Reger R, Hancock J [1980]. Coal miners exposed to diesel exhaust emissions. In: Rom W, Archer V, eds. Health implications of new energy technologies. Ann Arbor, MI: Ann Arbor Science Publishers, Inc., pp. 212-231.

Sydbom A, Blomberg A, Parnia S, Stenfors N, Sandström T, Dahlén SE [2001]. Health effects of diesel exhaust emissions. Eur Respir J 17(4):733-746.

Ulfvarson U, Alexandersson R [1990]. Reduction in adverse effect on pulmonary function after exposure to filtered diesel exhaust. Am J Ind Med 17(3):341-347.

Wichmann HE [2007]. Diesel exhaust particles. Inhal Toxicol 19 Suppl 1:241-244.

This page left intentionally blank

This page left intentionally blank

ACKNOWLEDGMENTS AND AVAILABILITY OF REPORT

The Hazard Evaluations and Technical Assistance Branch (HETAB) of the National Institute for Occupational Safety and Health (NIOSH) conducts field investigations of possible health hazards in the workplace. These investigations are conducted under the authority of Section 20(a)(6) of the Occupational Safety and Health Act of 1970, 29 U.S.C. 669(a)(6) which authorizes the Secretary of Health and Human Services, following a written request from any employer or authorized representative of employees, to determine whether any substance normally found in the place of employment has potentially toxic effects in such concentrations as used or found. HETAB also provides, upon request, technical and consultative assistance to federal, state, and local agencies; labor; industry; and other groups or individuals to control occupational health hazards and to prevent related trauma and disease.

Mention of any company or product does not constitute endorsement by NIOSH. In addition, citations to websites external to NIOSH do not constitute NIOSH endorsement of the sponsoring organizations or their programs or products. Furthermore, NIOSH is not responsible for the content of these websites. All Web addresses referenced in this document were accessible as of the publication date.

This report was prepared by Marie A. de Perio and Kenneth W. Fent of HETAB, Division of Surveillance, Hazard Evaluations and Field Studies. Eileen Birch of the Division of Applied Research and Technology provided us with modified cyclones and helped us interpret the elemental carbon sampling results. Industrial hygiene equipment and logistical support was provided by Donald Booher and Karl Feldmann. Health communication assistance was provided by Stefanie Evans. Editorial assistance was provided by Ellen Galloway. Desktop publishing was performed by Greg Hartle.

Copies of this report have been sent to employee and management representatives at the rail yard, the state health department, and the Occupational Safety and Health Administration Regional Office. This report is not copyrighted and may be freely reproduced. The report may be viewed and printed at http://www.cdc.gov/niosh/hhe/. Copies may be purchased from the National Technical Information Service at 5825 Port Royal Road, Springfield, Virginia 22161.

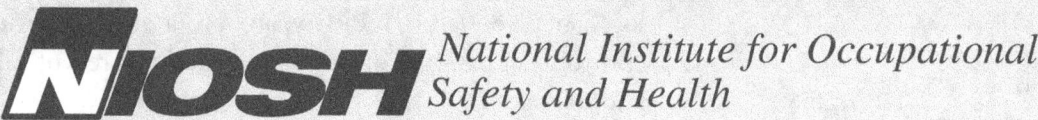

National Institute for Occupational Safety and Health

Delivering on the Nation's promise: Safety and health at work for all people through research and prevention.

To receive NIOSH documents or information about occupational safety and health topics, contact NIOSH at:

1-800-CDC-INFO (1-800-232-4636)

TTY: 1-888-232-6348

E-mail: cdcinfo@cdc.gov

or visit the NIOSH web site at: **www.cdc.gov/niosh.**

For a monthly update on news at NIOSH, subscribe to NIOSH eNews by visiting **www.cdc.gov/niosh/eNews.**

SAFER • HEALTHIER • PEOPLE™